ISBN 978-1-990666-88-9

TABLE OF CONTENTS

Salmon With Brown Sugar And Mustard

Ingredients:

- ¼ cup of Dijon mustard

- ¼ cup of dark brown sugar

- ½ a tablespoon of salt

- ½ tablespoon of ground pepper

- 1 side salmon about 3 pounds (cut into 8 fillets)

- Tablespoon of extra-virgin olive oil

- 1 large shallot

- ¼ cup of red-wine vinegar

- 1 lemon

Directions:

1. Heat your oven to 400 degrees and add salt and pepper to the salmon fillets.

2. Place the salmon fillets skin-side down on a lightly oiled, foil-lined baking sheet.

3. Make a mixture of Dijon mustard and brown sugar to the degree of spicy-sweetness that pleases you Slather the tops of the fillets with the mustard and brown sugar glaze and slide them into the top half of your oven.

4. Roast for about 12 minutes and serve.

Tuna Patties

Ingredients:

- 2 tablespoons of butter
- 3 tablespoons of all-purpose almond ground flax meal
- 1 cup of evaporated milk
- 5 ounces of light tuna in water
- ½ cup dry bread crumbs
- 1 green onion, finely chopped
- 2 tablespoons lemon juice
- ½ teaspoon salt
- ¼ teaspoon pepper
- Oil for frying

Directions:

1. In a small saucepan, melt butter over medium heat. Stir in almond ground flax meal until smooth; gradually whisk in milk. Bring to a boil, stirring constantly. Cook and stir until thickened, then remove from heat.

2. Transfer to a small bowl and let it cool down. Stir in tuna, 1/3 cup bread crumbs, lemon juice, salt and pepper. Refrigerate, covered, at

least 30 minutes. Place remaining ½ cup bread crumbs in a shallow bowl. Drop 1/3 cup tuna mixture into crumbs.

3.   Gently coat and shape into a ½ inch thick patty. In a large pan, heat oil over medium heat. Add tuna patties in batches and cook until golden brown, 2-3 minutes on each side. Place them on paper towels to drain and serve.

Chicken Wings

Ingredients:

- 2 tsp white wine vinegar

- 3 cloves garlic, minced

- ¼ tsp sea salt

- 2 lbs chicken wings

- 2 tbsp sesame oil

- ¼ cup tamari sauce

- 1 tbsp ginger powder

Directions:

1. Preheat oven to 400°F.
2. In a large container whisk together the ginger powder, sesame oil, salt, tamari sauce, vinegar, and garlic.
3. Add the wings to the mixture and stir to coat.

4. Place the wings on a lined baking sheet and bake for 30-35 minutes until golden and crispy.

5. If you want it crispier, turn on the broiler for a few minutes. Enjoy!

Baked Garlic Ghee Chicken Breast

Ingredients:

- 2 cloves garlic, chopped

- 1 tsp sea salt

- 1 tsp chives, diced

- 1 chicken breast

- 1 tsp garlic powder

- 1 tbsp ghee

Directions:

1. Preheat oven to 350°F.
2. Place the chicken breast on a piece of foil.
3. Season with sea salt, garlic powder, chopped fresh garlic. Top with ghee and rub everything into the chicken breast.
4. Wrap the chicken breast in the foil and place on a baking tray.

7

5. Bake for 30 minutes, or until chicken breast is cooked through, with a meat thermometer reading above 165°F.

6. Serve with more salt and ghee to taste. Cut the chicken breast into slices and sprinkle diced chives on top.

Tuna Muffins

Ingredients:

- ¼ cup sour cream

- 2 large eggs

- ¼ cup scallion, chopped

- 1 tablespoon fresh parsley, chopped

- 1 (7-ounce) can water-packed tuna, drained

- 3 ounces sharp cheddar cheese, shredded

- ¼ cup mayonnaise

- Salt and freshly ground black pepper, to taste

Directions:

1. Preheat the oven to 350 degrees F. Grease 6 cups of a muffin tin.
2. In a bowl, add all the Ingredients: and mix until well combined.

3. Place the muffin mixture into the prepared muffin cups evenly.

4. Bake for about 25-30 minutes or until top becomes golden brown.

5. Remove the muffin tin from the oven and place onto a wire rack to cool for about 10 minutes.

6. Invert the muffins onto a platter and serve warm.

Chicken & Bacon Waffles

Ingredients:

- 1 cooked bacon slice, crumbled

- 1/3 cup Pepper Jack cheese, shredded

- 1 teaspoon powdered ranch dressing

- 1 egg, beaten

- 1/3 cup cooked chicken, chopped

Directions:

1. Preheat a mini waffle iron and then grease it.
2. In a medium bowl, place all Ingredients: and with a fork, mix until well combined.
3. Place half of the mixture into preheated waffle iron and cook for about 3-4 minutes or until golden brown.
4. Repeat with the remaining mixture.
5. Serve warm.

Bacon On The Grill

Ingredients:

- 1 pound lean thick-cut bacon

- aluminum foil

Directions:

1. Preheat an outdoor grill for medium-low heat.
2. Line a large rimmed baking sheet with aluminum foil.
3. Place a cooling rack on top. Place bacon on rack, making sure no pieces are overlapping.
4. Place baking sheet on the grill grate, close the lid, and cook for 12 minutes or until desired doneness.
5. Transfer bacon to a paper towel-lined plate to absorb excess grease.

Flank Steak Marinade

Ingredients:

- 1 tablespoon granulated garlic

- 2 teaspoons honey

- 1 teaspoon onion powder

- 1 teaspoon ground white pepper

- ½ teaspoon grated fresh ginger

- ¾ cup soy sauce

- ¼ cup Worcestershire sauce

- 3 tablespoons fresh lemon juice

- 2 tablespoons sesame oil

Directions:

1. Mix soy sauce, Worcestershire sauce, lemon juice, sesame oil, granulated garlic, honey,

onion powder, white pepper, and ginger together in a bowl.

2. Transfer to a 1-gallon resealable plastic bag.

Breakfast Sausage Patties

Ingredients:

- ¼ tsp sage (dried)

- ½ tsp ground black pepper

- ½ tsp red pepper flakes

- 8 oz fresh ground pork

- 2 tbsp chicken stock

- ½ tsp thyme (dried)

Directions:

1. Using your hands, carefully combine all Ingredients: in a mixing bowl.
2. Fold a sheet of waxed paper in half.
3. Divide the sausage mixture into eight 2 - tablespoon portions and roll them into balls using your palms.

4. Place the balls on the waxed paper, fold over, and press down to compress the balls into patties.
5. Coat a non-stick skillet with cooking spray.
6. Cook the patties over medium-high heat for 10 minutes, turning halfway.
7. The sausage should cook until the internal temperature reaches 160°F.
8. Serve, and enjoy. Store any leftovers in the fridge.

Feta Chicken Patties

Ingredients:

- 6 oz feta (crumbled)

- 1 tbsp ground oregano

- ¼ tsp salt

- 1 lb ground chicken

- ¼ tsp garlic powder

Directions:

1. Preheat the grill or broiler.
2. Mix all of the Ingredients: together in a large mixing bowl.
3. Using your hands, roll the mixture into 4 equal-sized balls.
4. Press down on the balls with a decent amount of pressure to flatten them into formed patties.

5. Repeat this method until you have 4 chicken patties.

6. Grill or broil the patties until their internal temperature reaches 165°F or cook them for about 7 to 8 minutes per side. Make sure they are cooked throughout.

7. Enjoy them as part of a meal, snack, or on the go.

Parmesan Tuna Patties

Ingredients:

- 2 tbsp ground flax meal

- ½ tsp garlic powder

- ½ tsp onion powder

- ½ tsp salt

- 1 can of tuna (6 oz)

- 1 tbsp reduced fat/sugar mayonnaise

- 1 large egg

- 2 tbsp Parmesan cheese (finely grated)

Directions:

1. Drain the tuna until most of the water has been drained away.

2. Mix all the Ingredients: together in a medium-sized bowl, shape them into patties with your hands, and then put them in the oven.

3. Use about 1/4 cup of the mix for each cake. Place a skillet on medium-high heat and spray it with cooking spray before cooking, then stir.

4. Place the patties in the pan.

5. Once the burgers are in the pan, lightly press down with a fork to set each 2 .

6. Each 2 should be fried for a few minutes on each side until the edges are brown.

7. Do the same on the other side. They should cook quickly.

8. To serve them, take them out of the skillet and let them cool down for a few minutes before you do anything else.

9. You want to make sure they are completely cool before you put them in the fridge,

Chicken Gizzards And Broth

Ingredients:

- 1 tsp sea salt

- ¼ tsp ground black pepper

- 4 cups water

- 1 lb chicken gizzards (cut into quarters)

- 2 tbsp ghee

- 1 medium onion (chopped)

- 2 cloves garlic (chopped finely)

Directions:

1. Saute onions, garlic, and gizzards in your pressure cooker with the sauté setting.
2. When it's d2 cooking, add your water to the mixture.

3. Make sure to stir it from time to time. Make sure the lid is on.

4. The dish should be d2 in about 25 minutes at a high pressure.

5. It should be able to depressurize naturally before you open it.

6. The dish should be topped with chives and/or chive blossoms (optional).

Keto Chicken Liver Pate Recipe

Ingredients:

- 2 cloves garlic minced

- 1 tablespoon parsley minced

- ½ teaspoon salt

- ¼ teaspoon ground black pepper

- ½ pound chicken livers

- ½ cup butter or duck fat for dairy free

- 1 medium shallot minced

Directions:

1. Trim the chicken livers and remove any sinew. Kitchen scissors work well for this.

2. Melt a tablespoon of butter in a skillet over medium heat. Add garlic and shallots. Cook for 1-2 minutes until fragrant.

23

3. Add chicken liver to the pan. Pan-fry the first side until golden brown, flip them over for the second side, about 5-7 minutes total. Add parsley in the last minute of cooking.
4. Remove from heat and cool enough to add to a food processor. Add remaining butter and season with salt. Puree until smooth.
5. Pour into ramekin dishes or a container and chill for 4 hours or overnight to set.

Classic Beef Liver Pate

Ingredients:

- 1/2 teaspoon salt

- 1/2 teaspoon ground black pepper

- 2 tablespoons heavy whipping cream optional, preferably raw

- 1/2 pound beef liver

- 6 tablespoons grass-fed butter divided

- 2 cloves garlic finely minced

- 2 teaspoons dried thyme

Directions:

1. Melt 3 tablespoons of the butter in a skillet.
2. Add finely minced garlic and cook on medium-high until translucent, 3-4 minutes.

3. Meanwhile, trim the connective tissue off of the liver and slice to thin strips.

4. Add beef liver to pan, increase to high heat.

5. Sprinkle with thyme, salt, and pepper. Sear liver for 60 seconds on each side.

6. Remove liver from heat and let cool, about 5 minutes.

7. Transfer to a food processor or blender and puree until smooth.

8. While blending/pureeing, add the remaining butter and cream (if using).

9. Add more salt and pepper to taste, if desired.

10. Once the mixture is completely smooth, remove from blender and put in ramekins or a glass container and cover tightly.

11. Chill in the fridge for at least 4 hours or overnight (preferred) to harden and let flavors meld.

12. Serve with cucumber, celery, bacon or just a spoon.

Classic Carnivore Club Sandwich

Ingredients:

For the Duck Fat Mayonnaise:

- 2 tbsp apple cider vinegar

- 1 tsp Dijon mustard

- 1/4 tsp sea salt

- 1 cup duck fat

- 1 egg

- 2 egg yolks

- 1 tbsp fresh lemon juice

For the Carnivore Sandwich Bread:

- 5 oz pork rinds

- 1/4 cup grass-fed ghee (or butter)

- 1 tsp sea salt

- 8 eggs

- 1 lb raw ground pork

For the Club Sandwiches:

- 10 slices bacon

- 1 family size pack ham

- 1 family size pack turkey

- 1 block raw cheese

Directions:

1. Make the Duck Fat Mayonnaise.
2. Follow this recipe. Store the mayo in the fridge in an airtight container (or a condiment squeeze bottle, if you prefer) until you're ready to use it.
3. Make the Carnivore Sandwich Bread.

4. Follow this recipe. Note: if you can't tolerate pork, make Carnivore Sandwich Bread [Beef Version] instead.

5. Once done, allow the bread to rest on the countertop or on a cooling rack.

6. Once cooled, slice the bread into 1-inch thick slices (or whatever thickness you prefer), and set aside.

7. Cook the bacon.

8. In a cooking pan or in the oven, cook all of the bacon as you normally do.

9. Once done, set the bacon aside on a plate to cool.

10. Put it all together.

11. Toast the slices of bread, if preferred.

12. Drizzle the mayo on the insides of both ends of the bread.

13. Stack the ham, raw cheese, turkey, and bacon on top of the bottom slice of bread, and top with the other slice of bread.

14. If preferred, cut each sandwich in half. Place toothpicks in the half-sandwiches to hold the pieces together.
15. Serve, savor, and enjoy!
16. Store in an airtight container in the fridge for 1-2 days.

Carnivore Fried Chicken Strips

Ingredients:

- 6 oz pork cracklings (the equivalent of 2 4505 bags; pork rinds are find, but pork cracklings work better)

- 2 eggs

- 1.5 lbs chicken thighs

- Sea salt (to taste)

Directions:

1. Make the breading.
2. Take the pork cracklings* and blend them until they reach the consistency of an oily powder.
3. *Note: Pork rinds will work too, however, I could not achieve as thick of a breading layer with pork rinds.

4. Place the pork crackling powder in a medium-sized bowl.

5. Prepare the chicken strips.

6. Cut the chicken thighs into strips. I cut mine into strips that were about 4 inches long and 1/2-1 inch wide, but you can cut yours into whatever size you prefer.

7. Make the fried chicken.

8. Beat two eggs in a small bowl.

9. Dip each chicken strip into the egg mixture. Once fully coated, immerse it into the pork crackling powder and roll it around until it's fully coated with a thick layer. The powder will be oily and should stick together. Make sure the breading layer is thick.

10. Place the coated chicken strips onto a parchment paper-lined baking sheet. Salt them liberally.

11. Bake for 20 minutes at 400 degrees, flip, then bake for another 20-25 minutes. The coating

should be hard to the touch and crunchy when the chicken strips are finished. I made these in my air fryer and the 20 min-20 min at 400 degrees worked well.

12. Serve and enjoy! Make some Onion-Free Guacamole, Honey Mustard, or Duck Fat Ranch Dressing for dipping.

13. If you plan on saving them for later, store them in an airtight container in the fridge for 2-3 days.

Slow Cooker Beef Bone Broth Recipe

Ingredients:

- 2 medium carrots chopped

- 2 sprigs rosemary

- 1 clove garlic

- 1/4 cup raw apple cider vinegar lemon or lime juice

- 6 pounds beef bones

- 1 medium onion quartered

- 3 ribs celery chopped

Directions:

1. Preheat the oven to 350°F (177°C). Placing the b2 s in a roasting pan or baking dish. Roast for about 20 minutes, until golden brown.

2. Add all vegetables and herbs to the bowl of the slow cooker. Arrange b2 s on top of the vegetables. Cover all ingredients with water. Leave about 1-inch of space from the water line to the top of the slow cooker. Stir in the vinegar.

3. Cover with a lid. Cook on low for 18 to 24 hours.

4. Skim off any scum that rises to the top. Once cool enough to handle, strain the broth through a strainer and ladle into glass jars for storage.

5. B2 broth keeps in the fridge for up to one week, best if used in 3-5 days. It will freeze well for up to 3 months.

Easy Fish Stock Recipe

Ingredients:

- ¼ cup parsley chopped

- 6 sprigs thyme

- 4 whole black peppercorns

- 1 bay leaf

- 4 pounds fishbones with heads

- 2 tbsp butter

- 1 medium onion thinly sliced

- ½ cup dry white wine

Directions:

1. Heat the butter in a stockpot. Sauté the onions for 5-7 minutes, until slightly translucent.

2. Add the white wine and all remaining ingredients. Submerge all contents with water by 2-inches.

3. Bring water to a simmer, then reduce it to a very light simmer. Cook over this heat for 30 minutes. Skim off any foam or scum that rises to the surface.

4. Strain the stock through a fine-mesh strainer or cheesecloth.

5. Best served or used immediately. It will keep well in the fridge for up to a week.

6. Transfer to freezer-safe containers for long-term storage and save in the freezer for up to 3 months.

Roll-Ups With Cheese And Meat

Ingredients:

- 4 cooked turkey slices

- 4 cheese slices

Directions:

1. Place turkey slices on a serving plate and set aside.
2. On each, place a piece of cheese.
3. Place the roll with the seams facing down. If desired, secure with a toothpick before serving.

Marrow Roasted

Ingredients:

- 8 b2 marrow halves,

- To taste freshly ground pepper

- Flakes of salt

Directions:

1. Place the b2 marrow halves on a rimmed baking sheet with the marrow facing up.

2. Preheat oven to 350°F and bake for 20 to 25 minutes, or until crisp and golden brown. The majority of the fat will be expelled.

3. Serve with a pinch of salt and pepper to taste.

Carnivore Lemon Cheesecake

Ingredients:

Cheesecake

- 2 tbsp melted butter

- 1/2 tsp lemon extract

- 1/2 tsp vanilla extract

- zest of 1 fresh lemon OR 1 tsp dried lemon rind

- 2 bricks firm cream cheese (8 ounces each)

- 2 eggs

- 1/4 cup sour cream

- optional 2 tbsp SoNourished monkfruit sweetener

Topping

- 3/4 cup heavy cream

- 1/4 tsp vanilla extract

- fresh lemon zest (optional)

Directions:

Crockpot

1. Line your springform pan with plastic wrap.

2. Prepare batter by placing all ingredients in a mixing bowl and using an electric mixer, mix until smooth

3. Pour batter in the springform pan

4. Place a trivet (I used my InstantPot one!) in the bottom of the crockpot. Or use canning jar rings or rolled up tin foil, you want to elevate the pan above the water.

5. Pour 1 cup water in bottom of crockpot

6. Place pan on top of trivet. Cover the top of crockpot with paper towels to prevent water

dripping onto your cheesecake, then place lid over that.

7. Cook on high for 2 hours, then turn off crockpot and let sit for 1 hour.

8. Remove the cheesecake, keep it in the pan but cover in foil or plastic wrap and place in fridge overnight.

9. The next day, release the cheesecake from the pan onto a serving platter.

10. Whip the heavy cream with vanilla and smooth over top of the cheesecake.

11. Sprinkle with a little lemon zest (optional)

Instant pot

12. Line the springform pan with parchment paper to cover the bottom and sides, unless you have the silic2 springform pan.

13. The cheesecake batter instructions are the same.

14. Pour 1 1/4 cups water into the instant pot.

15. Place your trivet with lifters at the bottom of the Instant pot.
16. Cover the cake pan with a layer of foil. Place your foil covered cake pan on the trivet and lock the Instant Pot lid into place.
17. Select the Manual button and adjust cooking time to 30 minutes.
18. When cook time is complete, allow the pressure to release naturally for 15 minutes. Remove the cheesecake and allow to cool on the counter for another 15 minutes.
19. Transfer cheesecake to the fridge overnight (or minimum 4 hours).
20. Garnish with unsweetened whipped cream and lemon zest (optional)

Skillet Eggs With Thyme

Ingredients:

- ½ teaspoon kosher salt

- ¼ teaspoon freshly ground black pepper

- 1 sprig fresh thyme

- 1 tablespoon olive oil

- 1 tablespoon salted butter

- 4 eggs

Directions:

1. In a medium-sized pan, melt the oil and butter over medium heat until they start to sizzle.
2. This is how you should carefully crack each egg into the skillet.
3. You want to make sure the yolks aren't broken.

4. Eggs with salt and pepper are on top of thyme.

5. Cook for 112 minutes if you want runny eggs or 212 minutes if you want a firmer yolk.

6. Turn the heat down and cover. Remove the thyme sprig and serve right away.

Herby Chicken Omelet

Ingredients:

- ½ teaspoon freshly ground black pepper

- 2 tablespoons salted butter

- ⅓ cup grated mozzarella cheese

- 6 baby spinach leaves

- 2 ounces cooked chicken, shredded

- 4 eggs

- 1 egg yolk

- ½ teaspoon dried oregano

- ½ teaspoon ground thyme

- 1 teaspoon kosher salt

Directions:

1. Mix the eggs, egg yolk, oregano, thyme, salt, and pepper in a bowl.

2. Melt the butter in a nonstick pan over medium heat.

3. Add the egg mixture, let it cook for a minute, and then stir it into the food. Sprinkle the omelet with cheese, spinach, and chicken.

4. Turn down the heat to medium-low, cover, and cook for about 3 or 4 minutes, until the eggs are set, then remove the lid and serve.

5. Cut the omelet into 3 equal parts, slide them onto 3 separate plates, and eat them up! A good tip is to add some pickled jalapeno peppers at the end if you want to add a little heat.

Friendly Lemon Cheesecake

Ingredients:

Cheesecake

- 1/2 tsp vanilla extract

- zest of 1 fresh lemon OR 1 tsp dried lemon rind

- optional 2 tbsp SoNourished monkfruit sweetener

- 2 bricks firm cream cheese (8 ounces each)

- 2 eggs

- 1/4 cup sour cream

- 2 tbsp melted butter

- 1/2 tsp lemon extract

Topping:

- 1/4 tsp vanilla extract

- fresh lemon zest (optional)

- 3/4 cup heavy cream

Directions:

Crockpot

1. Line your springform pan with plastic wrap.

2. Prepare batter by placing all ingredients in a mixing bowl and using an electric mixer, mix until smooth

3. Pour batter in the springform pan

4. Place a trivet (I used my InstantPot one!) in the bottom of the crockpot. Or use canning jar rings or rolled up tin foil, you want to elevate the pan above the water.

5. Pour 1 cup water in bottom of crockpot

6. Place pan on top of trivet. Cover the top of crockpot with paper towels to prevent water

dripping onto your cheesecake, then place lid over that.

7. Cook on high for 2 hours, then turn off crockpot and let sit for 1 hour.

8. Remove the cheesecake, keep it in the pan but cover in foil or plastic wrap and place in fridge overnight.

9. The next day, release the cheesecake from the pan onto a serving platter.

10. Whip the heavy cream with vanilla and smooth over top of the cheesecake.

11. Sprinkle with a little lemon zest (optional)

Instant pot

1. Line the springform pan with parchment paper to cover the bottom and sides, unless you have the silicone springform pan.

2. The cheesecake batter instructions are the same.

3. Pour 1 1/4 cups water into the instant pot.

4. Place your trivet with lifters at the bottom of the Instant pot.

5. Cover the cake pan with a layer of foil. Place your foil covered cake pan on the trivet and lock the Instant Pot lid into place.

6. Select the Manual button and adjust cooking time to 30 minutes.

7. When cook time is complete, allow the pressure to release naturally for 15 minutes. Remove the cheesecake and allow to cool on the counter for another 15 minutes.

8. Transfer cheesecake to the fridge overnight (or minimum 4 hours).

9. Garnish with unsweetened whipped cream and lemon zest (optional)

Pot Roast Recipe With Gravy

Ingredients:

- 2 teaspoons sea salt

- 3-6 cups beef broth

- 4 tablespoons ghee or butter divided

- 1 4-5- lbs. pot roast

Directions:

Stove top:

1. Preheat oven to 325 degrees. Salt the roast on all sides. Heat heavy bottomed pan that
2. has a lid, over medium-high heat and add 2 tablespoons of ghee.
3. When the pan is really hot, on the bottom brown each side of the roast for about 1-2 minutes.

4. When the pot roast is browned on both sides, add the broth until the pot roast is covered and
5. replace the lid and place in the oven.
6. Cook for 2-3 hours in the oven, while still covered, until fork tender. Remove it from the oven and set aside.
7. Put a small saucepan over medium heat and add 1.5 cups of the leftover broth and the remaining 2 tablespoon of ghee.
8. Stir the saucepan continuously for 5-6 minutes until the broth reduces and becomes thickened.
9. Place the roast on a serving plate and slice crosswise. Pour the thickened sauce over the pot roast.
10. Serve and enjoy.

Instant pot:

1. Turn on the saute function and melt the ghee.

2. Add the pot roast and sear it on each side for about 2 minutes each.
3. Add the broth until the meat is covered and lock the lid, making sure the vent is closed.
4. Cook on high heat for 90 minutes.
5. Let the pressure release naturally and make sure it is fork tender.
6. Place a small saucepan over medium heat and add 1.5 cups of the leftover broth from the Instant Pot and 2 remaining tablespoon of ghee.
7. Stir the saucepan continuously for 5-6 minutes until the broth reduces and becomes thickened.
8. Transfer the pot roast to a serving plate and slice it crosswise.
9. Pour the sauce over the pot roast.
10. Serve and enjoy.

Slow cooker:

1. Preheat frying pan to medium-high heat and then melt the ghee.

2. Add the pot roast and sear it on each side for about 2 minutes until it is browned.

3. Add the roast to the slow cooker and pour in the broth until it covers the meat.

4. Cook on high heat for 6 hours or until the roast is fork tender.

5. Place a small saucepan over medium heat and add 1.5 cups of broth and remaining 2 tablespoons of ghee.

6. Stir the saucepan continuously for 3-5 minutes until the broth reduces and becomes thickened.

7. Transfer the pot roast to a serving plate and cut into slices crosswise.

8. Pour the thickened sauce over the pot roast.

9. Serve and enjoy.

Easy Fish With Lemon Caper Sauce Recipe

Ingredients:

- Fish pieces, 2 pound

- Minced garlic, 3 tablespoon

- Minced ginger, 3 tablespoon

- Cilantro, 1 cup

- Olive oil, 3 tablespoon

- Chopped tomatoes, 2 cup

- Grated ginger, 3 tablespoon

- Salt, to taste

- Black pepper, to taste

- Caper powder, 2 teaspoon

- Onion, 2 cup

- Lemon juice, 1 cup

- Vegetable broth, 2 cup

- Smoked paprika, half teaspoon

Directions:

1. Take a pan.
2. Add in the oil and onions.
3. Cook the onions until they become soft and fragrant.
4. Add in the chopped garlic and ginger.
5. Cook the mixture and add the tomatoes into it.
6. Add the caper powder, lemon juice and fish.
7. Mix the fish so that the tomatoes and spices are coated all over the fish.
8. Bake the fish for fifteen minutes.
9. When your fish is d2 , add in the cilantro.
10. Your dish is ready to be served.

Easy Brazilian Fish Stew Recipe

Ingredients:

- Water, 2 cup

- Minced garlic, 3 tablespoon

- Minced ginger, 3 tablespoon

- Cilantro, half cup

- Olive oil, 3 tablespoon

- Chopped tomatoes, 2 cup

- Fish broth, 2 cup

- Onion, 2 cup

- Lemon juice, half cup

- Fish mince, half pound

- Powdered cumin, half tablespoon

- Pineapple cubes, 2 cup

- Smoked paprika, half teaspoon

Directions:

1. Take a pan.
2. Add in the oil and onions.
3. Cook the onions until they become soft and fragrant.
4. Add in the chopped garlic and ginger.
5. Cook the mixture and add the tomatoes into it.
6. Add the spices and fish mince.
7. Add in the broth and pineapple cubes.
8. Mix the Ingredients: carefully and cover your pan.
9. Add cilantro on top.
10. Your dish is ready to be served.

Perfect Pate

Ingredients:

- ½ teaspoon of pepper

- ½ teaspoon of dried thyme

- 3 tablespoon of apple cider vinegar

- 2 tablespoons of cream

- 6 tablespoons of butter

- ½ cup onion finely minced

- 1 clove garlic finely minced

- ½ lb. of chicken liver

- ½ teaspoon of salt

Directions:

1. In a medium size pan, melt 3 tablespoons of the butter.

2. Add the finely minced onion and garlic and cook on medium until translucent- 3-4 minutes.
3. Meanwhile, trim the connective tissue off of the livers.
4. Add the livers to the pan and sprinkle with salt, pepper, and thyme.
5. Brown livers for 6-10 minutes until cooked on the outside and barely pink on the inside.
6. Add the apple cider vinegar and cook until it thickens, 2-3 minutes.
7. Remove the pan from the heat and let it cool for about 5 minutes.
8. Put the livers in a blender and puree until smooth.
9. While blending/pureeing, add the remaining butter and cream if using.
10. Add more salt and pepper to taste, if desired.

11. Once mixture is completely smooth, remove it from blender and put in a glass container and cover tightly.

12. Put in the refrigerator overnight to harden and let the flavors meld.

Sautéed Kidneys In Red Wine Sauce

Ingredients:

- ½ medium onion, finely diced

- 1 cup of mushrooms, cleaned and sliced

- ¼ cup red wine

- Lb. lamb kidneys

- ¼ cup wine vinegar

- Tablespoons of butter

- Tablespoons of olive oil

- Salt and pepper to taste

Directions:

1. To prepare kidneys for cooking, first rinse and pat dry.

2. With a sharp knife, remove the outside membrane, cut in half, and remove any white fat and tubes from center.

3. Place in the bottom of a medium bowl, cover with cold water and ¼ cup of wine vinegar. Let it soak for half an hour.

4. Remove from solution, rinse and pat dry. In a pan, melt the butter and oil and lightly brown the kidneys.

5. Remove and set aside. Next, add the onion and mushrooms to the pan and cook, stirring frequently, until onion becomes near translucent.

6. Add the wine and cook for another minute or so. Return kidneys to pan heat through and serve immediately.

Bifteck Hache (French Hamburgers)

Ingredients:

For the burgers:

- 1 tbsp fresh thyme leaves

- ½ tsp salt

- ½ tsp pepper

- 1½ lb ground beef

- 4 tbsps ghee

- 1 onion, diced

- 1 egg

For the sauce:

- ½ cup beef stock

- 2 tbsps ghee

- ¼ cup parsley, chopped

65

Directions:

For the burgers:

1. Place 2 tbsps of ghee into a frying pan and cook half the diced onions until translucent, about 2-3 minutes.

2. Allow the onions to cool and add them with the oil in the pan to a mixing bowl with the egg, ground beef, salt, pepper, and thyme leaves.

3. Mix well and form 8 patties.

4. In a frying pan, cook the patties with 2 tbsps of ghee until both sides are well browned, about 5-6 minutes per side.

For the sauce:

1. Place the ghee into a frying pan and saute the remaining half of the onions, until translucent, about 2-3 minutes.

2. Add the beef stock and let cook until reduced, about 2-3 minutes. Add in the parsley.

3. Serve the sauce with the burgers.

Lemon Ghee Roast Chicken

Ingredients:

- ½ cup ghee

- 1 tbsp salt

- 4 lb whole chicken, remove giblets

- 1 lemon, zested, sliced

- 1 lemon, halved

Directions:

1. Preheat the oven to 350° F.
2. Combine lemon zest and ½ tbsp salt and rub all over the chicken.
3. Sprinkle ½ tbsp salt into the chicken cavity and stuff with lemon halves and ¼ cup of ghee.
4. Brush the remaining ghee on the outside of the chicken.

5. Place the chicken in a roasting pan and arrange the lemon slices around the chicken.

6. Roast for 1 hour 45 minutes. Using a meat thermometer, cook until the internal temperature of the meat is 165°F.

7. Let the chicken rest for about 10 minutes before slicing and serving.

Beef Waffles

Ingredients:

- ¾ cup cheddar cheese, shredded

- 2 cooked bacon slices, chopped

- 2 eggs, beaten

Directions:

1. Preheat a mini waffle iron and then grease it.
2. In a bowl, place all the Ingredients: and mix until well combined.
3. Place ¼ of the mixture into preheated waffle iron and cook for about 2½-3 minutes or until golden brown.
4. Repeat with the remaining mixture.
5. Serve warm.

Beef Burgers

Ingredients:

- 1 ounce mozzarella cheese, cubed

- 1 tablespoon unsalted butter

- 8 ounces ground beef

- Salt and freshly ground black pepper, to taste

Directions:

1. In a bowl, add the beef, salt and black pepper and mix until well combined.
2. Make 2 equal-sized patties from the mixture.
3. Place mozzarella cube inside of each patty and cover with the beef.
4. In a frying pan, melt the butter over medium heat and cook the patties for about 2-3 minutes per side.
5. Serve immediately.

Grilled Flank Steak

Ingredients:

- ½ teaspoon garlic powder

- ½ teaspoon onion powder

- ½ teaspoon cumin

- ½ teaspoon chili powder

- 1 (1 1/2-pound) flank steak

- 2 tablespoons extra-virgin olive oil

- 1 teaspoon salt

- 1 teaspoon freshly ground black pepper to taste

Directions:

1. Combine olive oil, salt, pepper, garlic powder, onion powder, cumin, and chili powder in a small bowl to make a paste.
2. Rub 1/2 of the paste on each side of the flank steak and wrap tightly with plastic wrap.
3. Refrigerate for at least 2 hours or overnight.
4. Preheat a gas grill for high heat and lightly oil the grate.
5. Sear the steak for 3 minutes, turning counter-clockwise once after 1 1/2 minutes to create grill marks.
6. Flip steak over and sear an additional 3 minutes.
7. Reduce flame to medium-high and continue to cook 5 minutes more for medium-well, or until desired temperature.
8. Remove steak from grill and let rest 10 minutes before slicing.

Broiled Mackerel

Ingredients:

- 1 tablespoon white sugar

- ½ tablespoon grated fresh ginger root

- 4 mackerel fillets

- ¼ cup soy sauce

- ¼ cup mirin (Japanese sweet wine)

Directions:

1. Rinse fillets, and pat dry with paper towels. In a medium bowl, mix together the soy sauce, mirin, sugar and fresh ginger.

2. Place fillets into the marinade, and let stand for at least 20 minutes.

3. Preheat your ovens broiler, or an outdoor grill for high heat.

4. Broil the fillets, basting occasionally, until the fish flakes easily with a fork, about 5 to 8 minutes.

5. Serve with a lemon slice or long white radish slice as a garnish.

Shrimp For The Grill

Ingredients:

For the seasoning:

- 1 tsp Italian seasoning

- ½ tsp cayenne pepper

- 1 tsp garlic powder

- 1 tsp sea salt

For the grill:

- 1 lb shrimp, peeled and deveined (jumbo)

- Canola oil for the grill

- 2 tbsp extra virgin olive oil

- 1 tbsp freshly-squeezed lemon juice

Directions:

1. Preheat a grill pan or an outdoor grill to high heat.

2. To cook the shrimp in the oven, preheat the broiler.

3. If broiling, line a baking sheet or pan with some foil and coat it with nonstick cooking spray.

4. In a medium-large mixing bowl, stir together the seasoning Ingredients:; garlic powder, salt, Italian seasoning, and cayenne.

5. Add the olive oil and lemon juice and stir until it forms a paste.

6. Add the shrimp and toss it thoroughly to coat. If you are using smaller shrimp, stack them onto metal skewers or wooden skewers that have been soaked in water for at least 1 hour.

7. Brush the grill or grill pan with the Canola oil.

8. Grill or broil the shrimp, just until they turn pink and opaque, for about 2 to 3 minutes on each side, turning once halfway through.

9. Serve immediately for the best results.

Hickory Turkey Burgers

Ingredients:

- 1 tsp parsley

- 1 tsp paprika

- 1 tsp cumin powder

- 4 tbsp liquid egg substitute or 2 large beaten eggs

- 1 lb ground turkey

- 1 dash salt

- 1 tsp liquid hickory flavored sauce (reduced sugar)

- 1 tsp garlic powder

Directions:

1. Preheat the grill or fire up some coals to get started.

2. Using a medium or large mixing bowl, add all of the Ingredients: together and mix them together thoroughly.

3. Using your hands, roll the mixture into four equal-sized balls.

4. Press down on the balls to form equal-sized patties without causing them to break apart.

5. Store them in the fridge for a few minutes to set, or carefully place them on the grill.

6. Cook them for about 5 minutes on each side to ensure that they are cooked throughout. Use a spatula to ensure that they do not break apart as you grill them.

7. Serve and enjoy immediately or save them for later.

Yummy Meatloaf

Ingredients:

- 2 hard-boiled eggs (sliced)

- sea salt and ground black pepper to taste

- 1 tsp crushed garlic

- lb ground beef

- 1 onion (finely chopped)

- 2 large eggs (beaten)

- 4 tbsp plain full-fat yoghurt

Directions:

1. The oven should be set to 350°F. Salt, pepper, and garlic are some things you can add to the chopped onion. You can also add yogurt.

2. Stir in the ground beef again. Spray a bread pan with non-stick spray.

3. Do not use oil or butter, which could make the dish too oily. Add the mixture and the sliced boiled eggs to the bread tin, then bake it in the oven.
4. The meatloaf should be cooked for an hour before you serve it. Slice the loaf after it has been on the counter for about 10 minutes so it can set.
5. The food can be served hot, or it can be frozen for another time.

Cocoa Crusted Pork Tenderloin

Ingredients:

- ½ tsp chili powder

- 1 tbsp butter

- 1 lb pork tenderloin (trimmed)

- 1 tbsp cocoa powder (unsweetened)

- 1 tsp instant coffee

- ½ tsp cinnamon powder

Directions:

1. The oven should be set to 400°F degrees.
2. In a bowl, mix together all of the spices. Preparing pork tenderloin: Take out the thin silver tendon running down the middle of the loin. Do this before cooking.

3. When cooking the tenderloin, rub it with a little bit of butter. Season the loin with the whole spice mix.

4. It is best to use a cast iron or heavy-bottomed pan to get the heat up. Spray with cooking spray that doesn't stick.

5. Place the tenderloin in the pan and cook it on both sides until it's brown and crispy.

6. It's time to put the pan in the oven. Roast for 15 minutes or until the inside temperature of the chicken reaches 145°F.

7. It's time to take the pan out of the oven. Place the meat on a cutting board and let it rest for about 5 minutes before cutting it.

8. Enjoy the food at any time or freeze it for later use.

Homemade Pemmican Recipe

Ingredients:

- 1 tablespoon salt

- 2 tablespoons herbs and spices optional

- 400 grams beef tallow melted

- 300 grams lean meat dried and ground

- 100 grams beef liver dried and ground

Directions:

1. Combine the dry meat, liver, and salt in a medium mixing bowl. Add optional herbs and spices, mix well.
2. Melt tallow in a double boiler over medium heat.
3. Pour over the dry Ingredients:. Stir well until thoroughly combined. Break apart all clumps.

Tallow should fully incorporate into the meat. If still crumbly, add more melted fat.

4. Spread the mixture evenly in an 8×8-inch baking dish and leave to harden at room temperature or place in the refrigerator for 30-60 minutes. Once firm, score into squares. Alternatively, you can roll the "dough" into balls with your hands.

5. Store pemmican in an airtight container in the pantry. If made correctly, it is shelf-stable and will never spoil. You may also store it in the refrigerator if that makes you more comfortable.

Bone Broth Recipe

Ingredients:

- 6 pounds beef b2 s

- ¼ cup raw apple cider vinegar optional

Directions:

1. Arrange the bones in a single layer in a large roasting tray and place them in the oven at 450°F (232°C) for about 20 minutes, until golden brown. NOTE: This step is optional and followed to affect the end flavor of the broth.
2. Place all the b2 s in a large stockpot.
3. Fill with enough water to fully cover the material.
4. Pour in optional vinegar.
5. Bring the water to a boil, then reduce down to a simmer.
6. Adjust the flame and pot lid to maintain a low simmer.

7. Cook for at least 18 hours, and up to 72 hours. I tend to pull my batch after about 24 hours.

8. Check periodically to ensure the water remains over the bones. Add extra water as needed.

9. Let the broth cool slightly. If a layer of scum or film appears over the top, skim it off with a slotted spoon.

10. Strain the broth through a fine-mesh strainer or cheesecloth.

11. Store in glass jars in the fridge for up to 5 days or in the freezer for longer.

Zero Carb Milkshake

Ingredients:

- 2 tablespoons powdered monkfruit blend sweetener

- 1/2 - 1 dropperful toasted marshmallow flavor or 1/2 teaspoon vanilla extract

- 1 cup ice

- 1 cup water

- 3 tablespoons heavy cream

Directions:

1. Add to a blender
2. To a blender, add ice, water, heavy cream, sweetener and flavoring. You can use any flavoring - either 1 dropperful of concentrated flavor drops or 1/2 teaspoon of flavor extract.
3. Blend and pour

4. Blend milkshake until smooth and pour into a glass.

Keto Gummy Worms

Ingredients:

- 1 packet sugar free flavored electrolytes

- 1/2 teaspoon powdered erythritol sweetener

- Food coloring, optional

- 1 cup water

- 3 tablespoons unflavored gelatin

- Gummy worm mold

Directions:

1. To a small microwave safe bowl, combine water, gelatin, electrolyte powder and sweetener. Whisk until mixed.

2. Meat mixture in microwave in until dissolved (1-3 minutes) or heat on the stovetop until boiling. Remove from heat.

3. Add 2-3 drops of food coloring if using. You can separate the mixture into multiple bowls to do different colors.

4. Using a pipette that comes with the mold, squirt gelatin mixture into each cavity of the mold. Refrigerate for 1-2 hours or until hardened. Remove from the mold. Store in the refrigerator.

Easy Slow Cooker Keto Carnivore Beef Stew

Ingredients:

- 1 large carrot chopped

- 1 large onion chopped

- 4 cloves garlic minced

- 2 tsp dried thyme

- 2 tsp salt

- 1 tsp ground black pepper

- 2 pounds beef marrow bones

- 2 pounds chuck roast cubed

- 2 tbsp beef tallow or other cooking oil

- 6 cups bone broth

- 8 ounce mushrooms quartered

- 2 cups cauliflower chopped

Directions:

1. Turn the slow cooker on low and place the marrow b2 s in the center of the insert.
2. Cube the roast. Heat tallow in a large skillet over high heat.
3. Arrange the meat in a single layer and sear evenly on all sides.
4. Cook in batches if needed. Once cooked, add to the pot.
5. Rinse and chop all vegetables. Gather the herbs.
6. Place everything all in the pot on top of the meat.
7. Pour broth over it all. Season with salt and pepper.
8. Cover and cook on low for 6-8 hours.

Keto Breakfast Casserol

Ingredients:

- 1 cup cheddar cheese shredded

- ¼ cup Parmesan shredded

- ½ teaspoon dried thyme

- ½ teaspoon salt

- ½ teaspoon ground black pepper

- 1 tablespoon grass-fed butter

- 1 medium onion diced

- 2 cloves garlic minced

- 1 pound chicken sausage

- 10 whole eggs

Directions:

1. Preheat the oven to 350°F (175°C).

2. Warm butter in a frying pan over medium heat.

3. Sauté the onion and garlic together for 5 minutes.

4. Remove the sausage from its casing and add to the pan also.

5. Break apart into smaller pieces and brown all sides evenly, about 8 minutes.

6. While the sausage browns, whisk 10 eggs in a large bowl. Mix in the cheese, thyme, salt, and pepper.

7. Transfer meat to an 8×8-inch (20×20 cm) glass baking or casserole dish.

8. Arrange in a single, even layer on the bottom.

9. Pour the egg mixture over the meat.

10. Gently jiggle or tap the dish so the egg can settle down around the meat.

11. Bake for 20 minutes, until eggs are set and top is golden brown.

12. Let rest 5 minutes before slicing and serving warm.

Meatballs With Pepperoni

Ingredients:

- 1 teaspoon pepper, or as desired

- 1/2 pound pepperoni pieces, ground or minced 2 eggs, whisked

- 2 pound beef or chicken ground

- 1 tsp salt (or to taste)

Directions:

1. In a mixing basin, add all of the Ingredients: and stir thoroughly.
2. Form the mixture into tiny balls and put on a baking sheet lined with parchment paper.
3. Preheat the oven to 350°F and bake the meatballs for 20-30 minutes, depending on their size.

4. While baking, rotate the balls a couple of times.

5. Alternatively, you may cook the meatballs in a pan with a lid.

6. Cook until thoroughly cooked. Switch the balls around a few times.

Burgers With Liver

Ingredients:

- Drain extra blood half teaspoon pepper half pound ground liver

- Grass-fed beef, 1 pound

Directions:

1. In a mixing bowl, combine all of the Ingredients: and mix with your hands.
2. Form the Ingredients: into 7-8 equal parts and form into patties.
3. Grill on both sides on a hot grill until desired d2 ness is attained, then serve.

Soup And Broth

Ingredients:

- Pork skin, 5 1/3 ounces (optional)

- 8 quarts water + additional water for blanching

- 1 1⁄4 pound of pork b2 s (no flesh)

- 1 pound pig trotters (just the leg section)

- 1 entire chicken's b2 s

Directions:

1. Cut the bigger b2 s into smaller pieces using a knife.
2. Blanch the b2 s as follows: Grab a big pot. Put the trotters and the rest of the b2 s in it. Fill the pan with enough water to cover the b2 s.
3. Preheat the saucepan to medium-high. Bring the water to a boil. 10 minutes of boiling Turn

off the heat. Take out the b2 s and set them aside.

4. Remove the water and thoroughly rinse the pot.

5. Using a sharp knife, remove any blood clots from the b2 s.

6. Return the b2 s to the pot with the pork skin. Fill it with 8 liters of water. Bring the water to a boil.

7. Reduce the heat and let it to simmer.

8. Scum will begin to float at first. Remove and remove the scum using a big spoon. Trim any extra fat as well.

9. Cover and cook for 12 to 15 hours on low heat. The stock would have shrunk in size and become thicker.

10. Turn off the heat. Strain into a big jar with a wire mesh strainer after it has cooled.

11. 5-6 days in the refrigerator Broth that isn't utilized may be frozen.

12. Heat well before serving. Serve with salt &
pepper to taste.

Garlic And Herb Pork Loin Chop

Ingredients:

- 1 teaspoon kosher salt

- ½ teaspoon freshly ground black pepper

- 1 teaspoon paprika

- ½ cup chicken broth

- 1 tablespoon freshly squeezed lemon juice

- 1 tablespoon heavy cream

- 3 fresh basil leaves, chopped

- 4 garlic cloves, minced

- 1 tablespoon fresh thyme

- 5 tablespoons salted butter, melted

- 4 (3-ounce) b2 less pork loin chops

Directions:

1. A small bowl is an excellent place to mix the herbs and butter. Then, set it aside.

2. Rub salt, pepper, and paprika all over the pork chops to make them taste good.

3. 3 minutes: Heat a cast-iron pan over high heat for 3 minutes, or until it starts to smoke, then turn off the heat. In a skillet, use a fork to put pork chops in the pan and cook them for 3 minutes on each side. Take a plate and put the pork chops on it. Then, set them aside.

4. It's time to get rid of some of the browned bits in the pan. Pour in the chicken broth and lemon juice, and stir for a minute or so to get rid of them. Add the cream and start until it's all mixed in.

5. Turn over the pork chops and pour the herb and butter mixture into the pan. For 5 minutes, turn the heat down to medium-low

and use a spoon to baste the pork chops a few times.

6. Turn off the heat, cover with aluminum foil, let sit for 10 minutes, then remove the foil and serve. Serve right away. TIP: To get the best results, take the pork chops out of the fridge and let them sit for 30 minutes before cooking them.

Lamb Kebabs

Ingredients:

- ¼ teaspoon freshly ground black pepper

- ¼ teaspoon garlic powder

- 1 teaspoon Italian Spice Blend

- 1 pound lamb leg steak, cut into

- 1-inch cubes

- ¼ cup avocado oil

- ½ teaspoon kosher salt

Directions:

1. Bowl or Zip-Top Bag: Put the lamb inside.

2. Marinate your chicken by putting it in a bowl and putting the avocado oil in it with the salt and pepper, garlic powder, and Italian spice mix. Overnight: Pour marinade over the lamb

106

and put the bag in the fridge. The next day, open the bag and take out the lamb.

3. Remove the lamb from the marinade and put the chunks on metal or wooden skewers to eat them.

4. Using a grill pan, cook the skewers, turning them a few times, until they reach 145°F inside, about 10 minutes. TIP: Mix this with Loaded Sour Cream to make it even better.

Triple Meat Keto Carnivore Chili

Ingredients:

- .5 tablespoon spicy chili powder

- .5 teaspoon black pepper

- 2 teaspoons salt

- 1 teaspoon molasses

- 1 bottle corona premier beer

- 1 pound beef short ribs

- 1 pound ground beef

- 1 pound beef chuck diced

- 2 cups onion chopped

- 3 cloves garlic minced

- 64 ounces diced tomatoes

- 32 ounces crushed tomatoes

- 2 tablespoons jalapeno chopped

- 1 tablespoon chili powder

Toppings:

- Shredded cheese

- Diced jalapenos

- Chopped onion

- Sour cream

- Avocado

Directions:

1. Add all ingredients except the meat to the crockpot.
2. Stir to combine and taste to adjust spices to your liking.
3. Add all meat and stir to combine.

4. Cook on low for 9 hours or on high for 6 hours.

5. Take out the short ribs and remove meat from bone.

6. Dice short rib meat and mix back into chili.

7. Serve with sour cream, cheese, avocado, diced raw onion, jalapenos or whatever other toppings you like.

Bacony Carnivore Womelettes

Ingredients:

- 1 slice bacon, raw

- 1 egg, large

- Splash maple extract, if desired

- Hefty pinch of any spices or flavorings you'd like, as desired

Directions:

1. Put the bacon in a blender or food processor and turn it on.
2. Once the bacon is mostly ground up, put the egg and any seasonings down the chute and continue to run the machine until liquified and well-incorporated. This is your womelette slurry.
3. Heat your mini-waffle maker, as per its Directions:.

4. Pour half the slurry in the waffle maker and put the lid on.

5. Cook until golden or to your desired level of d2 ness, about 3-5 minutes max.

6. Remove from the waffle maker and repeat steps 4 and 5 with the remaining slurry.

7. Enjoy warm however you like.

Chicken Salad Made Simple

Ingredients:

- 1 cup crumbled feta cheese

- 4 bacon slices

- 4 peeled and quartered hard-boiled eggs

- 1 gallon sour cream

- 4-5 halves of chicken breast

- To taste salt

- To taste pepper

Directions:

1. Place the chicken in a large stockpot. Fill the container with cold water. Season with salt.

2. Preheat the stockpot to medium. Cook until the chicken is cooked through. Using tongs,

remove the chicken and lay it on the cutting board. Chop or shred the meat.

3. Preheat a skillet over medium heat. Cook until the bacon is crisp.

4. Place on a plate lined with paper towels after removing with a slotted spoon. Chop into pieces when cool enough to handle.

5. Fold the chicken, bacon, and other Ingredients: together gently in a mixing bowl.

6. Chill before serving.

Easy Salmon Patties Recipe

Ingredients:

- Vegetable oil, 3 tablespoon

- Salt to taste

- Black pepper to taste

- Eggs, 3

- Chopped onions, 3 tablespoon

- Chopped garlic, 3 teaspoon

- Green onions, 4 tablespoon

- Bread crumbs, half cup

- Salmon meat, 3 cups

- Chopped fresh dill, 3 tablespoon

Directions:

1. In a large bowl add in the onions and the garlic.
2. Add in the rest of the Ingredients:.
3. Make round patties from the mixture.
4. In a pan heat the vegetable oil.
5. Fry your salmon patties.
6. Dish your patties out when the patties turn golden brown on both sides.
7. Add cilantro on top.
8. You can serve it with any sauce that you prefer.
9. Your dish is ready to be served.

Easy Shrimp Scampi Recipe

Ingredients:

- Smoked paprika, half teaspoon

- Water, 2 cup

- Minced garlic, 3 tablespoon

- Minced ginger, 3 tablespoon

- Cilantro, half cup

- Olive oil, 3 tablespoon

- Fish broth, 2 cup

- Turmeric powder, 2 teaspoon

- Onion, 2 cup

- Shrimp pieces, 2 cup

- Cherry tomatoes, 2 cup

- Pasta, 2 pack

Directions:

1. Take a pan.
2. Add in the oil and onions.
3. Cook the onions until they become soft and fragrant.
4. Add in the chopped garlic and ginger.
5. Cook the mixture and add the shrimps into it.
6. Add the spices.
7. Add in the broth.
8. Mix the Ingredients: carefully and cover your pan.
9. Boil your pasta according to the Directions: on the package.
10. When the shrimps are d2 , add in the cherry tomatoes.
11. Mix the pasta into the mixture.
12. Add cilantro on top.
13. Your dish is ready to be served.

Veal Kidneys Flambé

Ingredients:

- 2 cups of mushrooms

- 1 tablespoon of vinegar

- 1 cup of melted salted butter

- 1 tablespoon of cracked pepper

- ½ cup brandy, (warmed)

- 6 veal kidneys, trimmed and cut into thin slices

- 2 cups of milk for soaking

- ½ cup of shallots, peeled and finely chopped

- 1 cup cream

- Salt to taste

Directions:

1. Soak trimmed kidneys in milk at room temperature for about an hour.
2. Remove and pat dry. In a frying pan, sauté mushrooms and shallots in butter.
3. Remove to a heated platter and keep warm.
4. Add more butter to the pan and when it foams, sauté the kidney slices in batches.
5. Add the vinegar to the pan and then the brandy. Light the brandy and let it flambé.
6. When the flame disappears, add the cream and pepper.
7. Bring to the boil and let the sauce reduce a bit and season to taste with salt.
8. Serve the kidney slices on heated plates garnished with shallot-mushroom mixture and a spoonful of the sauce.

Oven-Baked Parmesan Garlic Wings

Ingredients:

- ½ tsp Italian seasoning

- ½ cup Parmesan cheese

- 1 tsp garlic powder

- ¼ tsp crushed red pepper

- ¼ tsp salt

- 6 lbs whole chicken wings

- 8 tbsp butter, melted

- 1 egg

Directions:

1. Preheat the oven to 425° F. Cut the wings into 3 sections.

2. Put the wings on a baking sheet with a metal rack on top. Cook for 15 minutes.
3. Make the sauce by by combining the cheese, butter, seasonings, and egg in a small bowl.
4. Don't worry about using a raw egg in the sauce; the wings will be hot enough.
5. Remove the wings from the oven and flip them over. Turn on the broiler and broil for 5 minutes. Flip again and broil for another 5 minutes. Keep flipping and broiling until they are d2 to your desired crispness. They should reach an internal temperature of 165°F.
6. Toss immediately in the sauce.
7. Garnish with extra cheese.

Crispy Indian Chicken Drumsticks

Ingredients:

- 3 tbsp garam masala

- ½ tbsp coconut oil

- 2 lbs chicken drumsticks

- 2 tbsps salt

Directions:

1. Preheat the oven to 450° F
2. Smear a large baking tray with coconut oil.
3. In a bowl, mix the garam masala and salt.
4. Pat the drumsticks dry.
5. Coat each drumstick with the mixture and lay on the baking tray.
6. Bake for 40 minutes. Serve immediately.

Lamb Burgers

Ingredients:

- 1 tablespoon fresh rosemary, chopped finely

- 1 tablespoon fresh parsley, chopped finely

- 2 teaspoons ground cumin

- Salt and freshly ground black pepper, to taste

- 2 pounds ground lamb

- 9 ounces Halloumi cheese, grated

- 2 eggs

Directions:

1. Preheat the grill to medium-high heat. Grease the grill grate.
2. In a large bowl, add all the Ingredients: and mix until well combined.
3. Make 10 equal-sized patties from the mixture.

4. Place the burgers onto the grill and cook for about 5-8 minutes per side or until d2 completely.

5. Serve hot.

Chicken Kabobs

Ingredients:

- 1 cup fresh basil leaves, chopped

- Salt and freshly ground black pepper, to taste

- 1¼ pounds b2 less, skinless chicken breast, cut into 1-inch cubes

- ¼ cup Parmigiano Reggiano cheese, grated

- 3 tablespoons butter, melted

- 2 garlic cloves, minced

Directions:

1. In a food processor, add the cheese, butter, garlic, basil, salt and black pepper, and pulse until smooth.
2. Transfer the basil mixture into a large bowl.
3. Add the chicken cubes and mix well.

4. Cover the bowl and refrigerate to marinate for at least 4-5 hours.

5. Preheat the grill to medium-high heat. Generously, grease the grill grate.

6. Thread the chicken cubes onto pre-soaked wooden skewers.

7. Place the skewers onto the grill and cook for about 3-4 minutes.

8. Flip and cook for about 2-3 minutes more.

9. Remove from the grill and place onto a platter for about 5 minutes before serving.

Fish In Foil

Ingredients:

- 1 teaspoon ground black pepper

- 1 fresh jalapeno pepper, sliced

- 1 lemon, sliced

- 2 rainbow trout fillets

- 1 tablespoon olive oil

- 2 teaspoons garlic salt

Directions:

1. Preheat oven to 400 degrees F (200 degrees C). Rinse fish, and pat dry.

2. Rub fillets with olive oil, and season with garlic salt and black pepper. Place each fillet on a large sheet of aluminum foil. Top with jalapeno slices, and squeeze the juice from the ends of the lemons over the fish. Arrange

lemon slices on top of fillets. Carefully seal all edges of the foil to form enclosed packets. Place packets on baking sheet.

3. Bake in preheated oven for 15 to 20 minutes, depending on the size of fish. Fish is done when it flakes easily with a fork.

Chicken Bone Broth

Ingredients:

- 6 cups water, or as needed to cover

- 2 tablespoons apple cider vinegar

- 1 tablespoon salt

- ½ tablespoon ground black pepper

- Aluminum foil

- 1 leftover chicken carcass, broken into pieces

- 1 onion, roughly chopped

Directions:

1. Preheat the oven to 450 degrees F (230 degrees C). Line a baking sheet with aluminum foil.

2. Place chicken bones onto the prepared baking sheet.

3. Place baking sheet in the preheated oven and roast bones for 30 minutes.

4. Gently transfer bones from the baking sheet into a large and heavy stockpot. Add onion and enough water to cover the bones by 2 inches. Add vinegar, salt, and pepper and bring to a boil over high heat. Reduce heat to medium-low and simmer, partially covered, leaving enough space for steam to escape, for 4 to 5 hours. Check occasionally for froth or foam that develops on top of the water, removing it with a large spoon.

5. Remove from the heat and let cool. Strain broth through a fine mesh strainer into a clean pot. Let cool completely. Store in the refrigerator and use within 5 days or freeze until ready to use.

Chicken Pops

Ingredients:

- ½ tsp turmeric

- ½ tsp paprika

- ¼ cup parsley leaves (finely chopped)

- 2 lemons (halved)

- 4 large chicken drumsticks, with the skin removed (about 4 ounces each)

- 3 cloves garlic (minced)

- 1 shallot (minced)

- 1 tbsp low-sodium soy sauce

- 1 tsp mustard

- ¼ tsp ground black pepper

Directions:

1. Mix together the first 8 Ingredients: along with the juice of half a lemon in a large mixing bowl.

2. Set aside about 3 tbsp of the mixture.

3. Preheat an outdoor grill to 400°F.

4. Place the chicken drumsticks on a cutting board. Using a sharpened chef's knife, cut the non-meat end around the b2 turning the leg toward the knife. (Optional: Using small kitchen pliers, pull out the white tendons and discard them.)

5. Holding the bony end of the leg with 2 hand, use your other hand to gently push the meat up and toward the flesh end to form a "lollipop." Remove the remaining flesh from the b2 by scraping it off with a knife.

6. Repeat the same technique with the rest of the drumsticks, placing each of them into the

bowl with the marinade mixture as you finish prepping them.

7. Place the marinated drumsticks on the preheated grill, along with the remaining 3 lemon halves (flesh side facing down).

8. After 10 minutes, remove the lemons from the grill and turn the drumsticks. Grill the chicken for another 10 to 13 minutes, until they reach an internal temperature of 165°F.

9. When the lemons are cool enough to touch, squeeze them into the remaining sauce.

10. Pour the sauce over the pops and enjoy while they are still nice and warm.

Beef Chuck Roast

Ingredients:

- 3 lb beef chuck (arm pot roast)

- 4 cloves garlic (peeled and halved)

- 1 tsp ground black pepper

Directions:

1. Preheat the oven to 400°F.

2. Secure the roast with cooking twine.

3. Make 8 slits of about ½ an inch each around the roast and insert half of a garlic clove into each cavity. Flavor with some fresh ground pepper and place it on a rack in a roasting pan.

4. Let it roast in the preheated oven for 20 minutes.

5. Reduce heat to 325°F and insert the meat thermometer into the roast.

6. Continue cooking for about 1 hour or until the roast is nice and tender. Do not overcook the roast, as it can become tough.

7. Remove it from the oven and loosely cover the roast with aluminum foil. Let it rest while covered for about 15 minutes before slicing or carving.

8. To serve, slice thinly against the grain, and use the pan drippings as gravy. If you wish to store it in the fridge, make sure that it cools down completely before putting it away.

Carnivore Freezer Pizza

Ingredients:

- 2 cups mozzarella cheese

- 2 cups diced bacon

- 1 low-carb or keto tortilla (large)

- 2 tbsp ranch dressing (reduced sugar)

- 12 oz ground beef (not lean)

- 1 serving pepperoni (13 pieces)

Directions:

1. The oven should be set to 400°F. A tortilla should be placed on a baking sheet that has been sprayed with cooking spray, like this: Ranch dressing: Add the ranch dressing, then spread it all over the tortilla surface.

2. As you keep adding the cheese and meat, pepperoni, and diced bacon, keep adding

more. Check to ensure that all Ingredients: are spread out evenly across the surface of the pizza so that they cover the whole thing.

3. It will take about 15 minutes for the cheese to melt and the toppings to get golden brown. The pizza should be in the oven when it's d2 . Serve it hot, or let it cool down for an hour and put it in the freezer.

4. Make sure the food is out of the freezer and put it in a 400°F oven for 5 to 10 minutes so it can warm up again

Easy Roast Beef

Ingredients:

- 1 tsp cracked black pepper

- 2 ½ lb top round beef roast

Directions:

1. The oven should be set to 400° F. When it's time to cook the meat, take it out of the fridge and let it come to room temperature for about 20 minutes.

2. It's best to dry the meat with paper towels to get rid of any water. Season the beef with black pepper, then rub the pepper on it. Pour some olive oil into a cast-iron skillet or a heavy oven-safe sauté pan and heat it up.

3. Do not add cooking spray or oil to the pan because grease is not needed at a moderate heat. In a pan, cook the meat on all sides. Then, move the pan into an oven.

4. For 50 minutes, roast it in a 350°F oven. The inside temperature should reach 125°F, which means it's d2 cooking.

5. It's time to take the meat out of the oven. Wrap the meat in foil and let it rest for 10 minutes before cutting into thin slices. Store for later use or enjoy all day long.

Slow Cooker Beef Bone Broth Recipe

Ingredients:

- 3 ribs celery chopped

- 2 medium carrots chopped

- 2 sprigs rosemary

- 1 clove garlic

- 1/4 cup raw apple cider vinegar lemon or lime juice

- 6 pounds beef b2 s

- 1 medium onion quartered

Directions:

1. Preheat the oven to 350°F (177°C). Placing the bones in a roasting pan or baking dish. Roast for about 20 minutes, until golden brown.

2. Add all vegetables and herbs to the bowl of the slow cooker. Arrange bones on top of the vegetables. Cover all Ingredients: with water. Leave about 1-inch of space from the water line to the top of the slow cooker. Stir in the vinegar.

3. Cover with a lid. Cook on low for 18 to 24 hours.

4. Skim off any scum that rises to the top. Once cool enough to handle, strain the broth through a strainer and ladle into glass jars for storage.

5. Bone broth keeps in the fridge for up to one week, best if used in 3-5 days. It will freeze well for up to 3 months.